Keto Diet for Beginners

Simple, Quick and Easy Recipes for Rapid Weight Loss: The Complete Instant Pot Ketogenic Diet Cookbook to Start Small and Lose 5+ Pounds in Days

Introduction

Welcome to the book, *"Keto Diet for Beginners: Simple, Quick and Easy Recipes for Rapid Weight Loss: The Complete Instant Pot Ketogenic Diet Cookbook to*

Start Small and Lose 5+ Pounds in Days." Many people make the mistake of thinking that successfully losing weight is all about working their butts off until they pass out from exhaustion. Thinking that they don't mind their diets – and are surprised that they aren't losing weight. Don't make the same mistakes as them.

You see, weight loss experts know something that the majority of the entire population of the world doesn't: that the greater chunk of successful weight loss is diet. Exercise helps speed up and maintain weight loss, but diet is what really makes losing weight possible.

The problem with most diets – at least what many people believe about them – is that losing weight means a diet of unpalatable foods. Nothing can be further from the truth. In this book, you will learn 19 delicious and easy-to-prepare ketogenic diet friendly recipes using your Instant Pot electric pressure cooker. By the end of this book, you'll have no more reasons not to eat right and lose weight. These recipes aren't just easy-to-prepare, but they're also delicious! If these aren't good enough to encourage you to eat right and lose weight, I don't know what will!

the information herein, either directly or indirectly. Respective authors own all copyrights not held by the publisher.

The information herein is offered for informational purposes solely and is universal as so. The presentation of the information is without a contract or any type of guarantee assurance.

The trademarks that are used are without any consent, and the publication of the trademark is without permission or backing by the trademark owner. All trademarks and brands within this book are for clarifying purposes only and are the owned by the owners themselves, not affiliated with this document.

Table of Contents

GREEN POT CHILI

4 Servings with 6 grams of carbs per serving

<u>Ingredients:</u>
- 1 ½ teaspoons of salt;
- ½ onion, chopped;
- ¼ cup of water;
- 2 jalapeño peppers chopped, with stems and seeds removed;
- 2 teaspoons of ground cumin;
- 3 poblano peppers chopped, with stems and seeds removed;
- 5 garlic cloves;
- 7 tomatillos, quartered and husked; and
- 8 pieces skinless, boneless chicken thighs.

For the Finishing:
- 1/3 packed cup of chopped cilantro leaves plus extra for garnishing; and
- Fresh squeezed juice of 1 lime.

<u>Directions:</u>

- Put the water, onions, poblanos, tomatillos, and jalapeños in the Instant Pot. Then spread out the salt, cumin, and garlic on top.
- Put the chicken thighs in and securely close the pot's lid.
- Use the high pressure setting to cook for 15 minutes. When done, release the pressure manually.
- After removing the lid, transfer the chicken thighs onto a cutting board so you can slice it into bite-sized pieces. Set them aside when done.
- Put the lime juice and the cilantro leaves in the pressure cooker and puree the mixture using an immersion blender. If you don't have one, just pour the remaining ingredients in a regular blender together with the cilantro leaves and lime juice and blend it.
- Set your Instant Pot to sauté mode and if you used a regular blender to puree the mixture, pour the mixture back into the Instant Pot.
- Place the cut chicken pieces back into the Instant Pot and allow it to boil in the pureed mixture – with occasional stirring - for up to 10 minutes or until the sauce turns thick.
- When done, remove from the pot to enjoy. If desired, use the extra cilantro to garnish.

WINE-BRAISED BEEF

This recipe is good for 6 servings with only 6 grams of carbs per serving.

<u>Ingredients:</u>

- 1 bay leaf;
- 1 cup beef broth plus extra in case needed;
- 1 cup red wine;
- 1 pound white button mushrooms, sliced;
- 1 tablespoon tomato paste;
- 1 yellow onion (large), spiralized;
- 2 peeled carrots, spiralized;
- 3 celery stalks, diced;
- 3 cloves of garlic, minced;
- 3 pounds of cubed beef round roast;
- 4 fresh sprigs of thyme;
- 5 bacon slices, chopped;
- Parsley for garnishing, chopped; and
- Pepper and salt to taste.

<u>Directions:</u>

- Cook the bacon in a big skillet heated over medium-high heat until they turn crispy. When done, transfer the bacon bits to a paper towel-lined plate.
- Season the beef cubes with salt and pepper. Put them in the hot skillet and arrange in a single layer. In case the skillet can't fit all the beef cubes in one layer, cook the beef cubes by batches.
- Sear the beef cubes on all sides for a total of 18 minutes, i.e., 3 minutes for each of the 6 sides.

- Next, place all the beef cubes inside your Instant Pot Cooker. Throw in the bacon slices, onions, celery, garlic, and mushrooms too. Cover the thyme sprigs and bay leaves with the mixture.
- Pour the wine and broth in, which should submerge the mixture up to ¾ of its height.
- Seal the pot's cover in and cook the mixture for 4 hours on high setting.
- Throw the spiralized carrot noodles in very quickly and immediately cover your Instant Pot again. Continue cooking for another hour, by the end of which your beef cubes will be so tender that you can easily pull them apart.
- Finally, stir the mixture one final time and remove the bay leaves before enjoying.

REUBEN'S POT SOUP

This recipe is good for 8 servings with only 4 grams of carbs per serving.

<u>Ingredients:</u>
- 1 ½ cups of sauerkraut;
- 1 cup of Swiss cheese, grated finely;
- 1 package of cream cheese (approximately 8 ounces), softened;
- 1 teaspoon fine salt;
- ½ teaspoon pepper, freshly ground;
- ¼ cup of onions, minced;
- 2 ½ cups of beef broth;
- 2 cups of corned beef, sliced thinly to look like noodles; and
- Fresh oregano for garnishing.

<u>Directions:</u>
- Inside a 6-quart Instant Pot, put the broth and the cream cheese and use a whisk to mix thoroughly.
- Put all the other ingredients in, tightly close the pot's lid, and close its vent. Use the pot's "SOUP" setting, which will automatically set the cooking time and the temperature.
- After the timer sounds off, manually release the pot's pressure using NPR. However, it may take up to 20 minutes for the pot's vent to completely open so be prepared to wait a bit.
- Enjoy with oregano sprig garnish.

POT BEEF CURRY

This recipe is good for 6 servings with only 8 grams of carbs per serving.

Ingredients:
- 1 pound of broccoli florets;
- 1 tablespoon of garlic powder;
- 1/2 cup of chicken broth;
- 14 ounces of canned coconut milk;
- 2 tablespoons of curry powder;
- 2 1/2 pounds of beef stew chunks;
- 3 zucchinis, sliced; and
- Salt for tasting.

Directions:
- Just put all the stew's ingredients in the Instant Pot and make sure that you mix the ingredients well and that the beef is at the bottom of the pot.
- Cook the stew for 45 minutes on high pressure via the pot's manual setting.
- After 45 minutes, turn the pot off and follow the manufacturer's instructions for releasing the pressure.
- After completely releasing the pressure, open the pot and mix the coconut milk in gently. If you want to, you can add more salt to taste before enjoying.

INSTANT POT CHICKENUFFALO SOUP

This recipe is good for 6 servings with only 4 grams of carbs per 1 cup serving.

Ingredients:
- 1 pound of chicken, cooked and shredded;
- 1 tablespoon of olive oil;
- ½ cup celery, diced;
- ½ cup of heavy cream, e.g., half-and-half;
- ½ onion, diced;
- 3 tablespoons of Buffalo sauce;
- 4 cups of chicken broth;
- 4 garlic cloves, minced;
- 6 ounces of cream cheese, cubed and at room temperature;

Directions:
- Use the "SAUTE" function of your Instant Pot to cook the celery and onion in oil for 5 to 10 minutes, with occasional stirring, until the onions turn brown and translucent.
- Mix the garlic in and continue sautéing for another minute or until the garlic smells fragrant. Turn the pot off.
- Put the Instant Pot's lid on and seal tightly before using the SOUP function to cook for 5 minutes. When done, naturally release the pot's pressure, which should take about 5 minutes. Revert to quick release and open the Instant Pot's lid.

- Scoop out 1 cup worth of the liquid without any chicken pieces from the pot and pour it inside a blender.
- Add in the cream cheese cubes and puree the mixture until you get a smooth textured mixture. When done, pour the mixture into the pot.
- Mix the heavy cream in and continue stirring until you get a smooth textured mixture.

CHICKEN HONEYAKIS

This recipe is good for 4 servings with 22 grams of carbs per serving.

Ingredients:
- 1 tablespoon of sesame seeds
- 1 teaspoon of fresh ginger, grated
- 1 teaspoon of sriracha
- 1/4 cup of low sodium soy sauce
- 2 cloves of garlic
- 2 tablespoons of honey
- 3 tablespoons of rice wine
- 8 chicken drumsticks without skins
- Scallions, chopped

Directions:
- Stir-fry your garlic, sriracha, ginger, and honey in rice wine and soy sauce for 2 minutes using your Instant Pot's sauté function.
- Put the drumsticks in your Instant Pot, cover it, and lock the lid to cook on high pressure for 20 minutes.
- Let the pot's pressure naturally dissipate after the 20-minute, high pressure cooking period.
- Once all the pressure has dissipated, mix the scallions and sesame seeds in before serving.

CHICKENUFFALO POT MEATBALLS

This recipe is good for 6 servings with less than 1 gram of carbs per serving.

<u>Ingredients:</u>
- 1 ½ pounds of ground chicken meat;
- 1 teaspoon of salt;
- 2 cloves of garlic, minced;
- 2 green onions, thinly cut;
- 2 tablespoons of ghee;
- ¾ cup of almond meal;
- 4 tablespoons more of ghee or butter;
- 6 tablespoons of hot sauce; and
- Green onions for garnishing, chopped.

Directions:
- Mix together the almond meal, chicken, minced garlic cloves, green onions, and salt in a big bowl. Combine these ingredients with your own hands but take care to avoid overworking the ground chicken meat.
- Use coconut oil or ghee to lubricate your hands and manually create 1 to 2-inch wide meatballs using the mixture.
- Put 2 tablespoons of ghee in your Instant Pot and set it to SAUTE.
- Brown the chicken meatballs in the pot by gently placing them in batches. Turn the balls every 60 seconds until the balls are evenly browned all over.

- As you're browning your meat, prepare your buffalo sauce. By heating together 4 tablespoons of butter or ghee and hot sauce on a stovetop or microwave until the butter or ghee has melted completely. Stir the melted mixture with a spoon.
- Once all the chicken meatballs have been browned, place them all back in the Instant Pot and pour the buffalo sauce evenly on them. Close the lid of the pot, ensuring the pressure valve is set to "SEALING" before setting the pot to "POULTRY" to cook the chicken buffalo meatballs for 15 to 20 minutes. Your Instant Pot will beep once it's done.
- If you're that hungry and want to eat your chicken buffalo wings as soon as possible, hit the "CANCEL" button and manually release the pot's pressure valve. Make sure your hands are safely away from where the steam is released from the Instant Pot. But if you can wait, your Instant Pot will automatically switch to "WARM" and the pressure will gradually be released.

HUNGARIAN GOULASH INSTANT POT STYLE

This recipe is good for 8 servings with only 8.33 grams of carbs per serving.

<u>Ingredients:</u>
- 1 ½ cups of chicken broth;
- 1 cup of chopped onion;
- 1 green pepper, sliced;
- 1 piece of bay leaf;
- 1 teaspoons of salt;
- ½ teaspoon of caraway seeds;
- ½ teaspoon of pepper;
- 2 cloves of garlic;
- 2 cups of daikon radish, cut into cubes;
- 2 pounds of beef stew meat, cut into cubes;
- 2 stalks celery, cut;
- 2 tablespoons of butter;
- 2 tablespoons of Hungarian paprika; and
- A 15-ounce can of diced tomatoes.

<u>Directions:</u>
- On a large sauté or frying pan, melt the lard or grease over medium heat and stir-fry your onions in it until they become translucent. Throw the paprika and garlic in and continue stir-cooking for 1 minute.
- Mix the cubed beef in and continue cooking until all their sides are browned. Throw in the salt, pepper, and caraway seeds, mix and transfer the pan's content to your 6-quart Instant Pot.

- Add in the radish, pepper, tomatoes, celery, broth, and bay leaf and stir the mixture thoroughly.
- Set your Instant Pot to "LOW" and its time to 6 hours and cook. If you want a shorter cooking time, set it to "HIGH" and cook for 4 hours.

NO-THAW-NEEDED GARLIC LEMON SALMON

This recipe is good for 4 servings with no carbs.

<u>Ingredients:</u>
- 1 ½ pounds salmon fillets, frozen;
- 1 tablespoon of melted coconut oil;
- 1 thinly sliced lemon;
- 1/8 teaspoon of black pepper;
- ¼ cup of lemon juice;
- ¼ teaspoon of garlic powder or 2 minced cloves of garlic for tasting;
- ¼ teaspoon of salt for tasting;
- ¾ cup of water; and
- A couple of fresh basil, dill, or parsley.

<u>Directions:</u>
- In your Instant Pot, pour the lemon juice and water. Throw the fresh herbs into the lemon water mixture in the pot and put the steamer rack inside the pot.
- Drizzle the coconut oil over your salmon and sprinkle with pepper, salt, and garlic powder to season.
- Lay your salmon pieces across the steamer rack inside the pot. Do not steam them stacked on top of one another as it will prevent them from cooking evenly. If they're stuck to each other, place the areas where they're joined together under running water to thaw just enough to separate them.

- Cover the pot with the lid, lock the cover, and put the valve in SEALING mode. Set the Instant Pot to MANUAL setting and cook for 7 minutes under high pressure.
- When done, switch your Instant Pot's valve to VENTING mode to release its pressure quickly.
- Remove cover and serve the salmon while warm.

CHICKEN SHREDDER IN A POT

This recipe is good for 20 servings with less than 1 gram of carbs per serving.

<u>Ingredients:</u>

- 4 pounds of chicken breast;
- 1/2 teaspoons of salt;
- 1/2 teaspoons of black pepper;
- 1 tablespoon of your favorite spices; and
- 1 cup of chicken broth.

<u>Directions:</u>

- Place the chicken breasts inside the pot and sprinkle with the Italian seasoning, salt, and black pepper to season. Pour the chicken broth around the chicken breasts.
- Close and lock your Instant Pot's lid. Use either the POULTRY or MANUAL setting, cook for 8 minutes (if the chicken breasts are already thawed or are fresh) or 13 minutes (if chicken breasts are still frozen).
- When the Instant Pot cooker stops, let it naturally release the pressure for at least 5 minutes. If you can't wait for more than 5 minutes, you can manually release the pressure after 5 minutes.
- Unplug the Instant Pot from the electrical outlet.
- Use 2 forks to manually shred the chicken breasts inside the Instant Pot. Doing so will allow you to shred the chicken while making sure it continues mixing with the tasty juices.

- Enjoy drained or with the juices. Either way, they're delicious! If you plan to save some for later, keep it with the broth so that it can retain its moisture.

INSTANT POT CHICKACCIATORE

This recipe is good for 4 servings (1 serving = 1 chicken thigh with ½ cup of sauce) with 10.5 grams of carbs per serving.

Ingredients:
- Salt and pepper for tasting;
- Olive oil spray;
- 4 skinless and boneless chicken thighs;
- 2 tablespoons of parsley or basil, chopped
- 14 ounces of crushed tomatoes;
- ¼ cup of red bell pepper, diced;
- ½ teaspoon of dried oregano;
- ½ cup of onions, diced;
- ½ cup of green bell pepper, diced; and
- 1 bay leaf.

Directions:
- Rub pepper and salt on both sides of the chicken pieces to season.
- Put the Instant Pot on SAUTÉ mode and spray the pot's inside with the olive oil. Brown both sides of the chicken pieces for a couple of minutes and set aside when done.
- Spray more olive oil and sauté the peppers and onions for about 5 minutes or until they turn soft.
- Pour the tomatoes on the vegetables and chicken in the pot. Then, mix the pepper, salt, bay leaf, and oregano in. Stir quickly, cover, and lock the lid.

- Cook using high pressure for 25 minutes before naturally releasing the pressure from the pot.
- Before serving, take the bay leaf out and use the parsley or basil to garnish.

OXTAIL SOUP

This recipe is good for 8 servings with 11 grams of carbs per serving.

Ingredients:
- Salt and pepper for tasting;
- 3 pieces of bay leaves;
- 3 1/2 pounds of oxtail of about 50% meat;
- 2 tablespoons of fresh lemon juice;
- 2 sprigs thyme;
- 2 sprigs rosemary;
- 2 medium-sized leeks, cut;
- 2 medium-sized celery stalks, cut;
- 2 cups of chopped green beans;
- 2 1/2 liters of water;
- 1/4 teaspoons of cloves, ground;
- 1/4 cup of ghee;
- 1 medium-sized rutabaga, diced; and
- 1 big can of unsweetened tomatoes.

Directions:
- Grease a big Dutch oven with ghee and heat it on medium-high heat.
- While heating your Dutch oven, use paper towels to pat-dry the oxtails. Sprinkle with salt and pepper on both sides to season.
- Brown the oxtails on all sides before placing them inside the Instant Pot. Close and lock the lid.
- Cook using your pot's high-pressure setting for 4 hours. Add the veggies within the last 60 minutes of cooking.

- Place the bay leaves, thyme, cloves, and rosemary in cheesecloth. Tie the cheesecloth using a kitchen string without wax. Doing this will enable you to easily remove these spices from the pot very easily after cooking. Put the cheesecloth in the pot before pouring the water and lemon juice in. When the mixture starts to boil, bring the heat to LOW to allow it to simmer for 3 more hours – with cover – or until the oxtail becomes so tender that the meat can fall off the bone.
- Use kitchen tongs to remove the oxtail from the pot to cool on a plate.
- While the oxtail's cooling down, cut and peel the rutabaga into inch-sized pieces. Put them in the pot to cook for another 10 minutes.
- Shred the meat once it becomes cool enough. You can keep the oxtail's gelatin part if you want to make bone broth for preparing other recipes later on.
- Mix the celery stalks, green beans, tomatoes, and leeks in, cover, and cook for another 15 minutes or until the rutabaga and beans turn soft.
- Place the shredded meat back in the pot and season with salt and pepper before serving.

INSTANT POT CORNED BEEF AND CABBAGE

This recipe is good for 4 servings with 9 grams of carbs per serving.

<u>Ingredients:</u>
- 5 cups of water;
- 3 1/2 pounds of corned beef brisket, with spices;
- 2 cups of baby carrots; and
- 1 small head of green cabbage cut into 8 wedges.

<u>Directions:</u>
- Drain and rinse the corned beef if you'll use cured corned beef. If not, no need to do so.
- Inside your Instant Pot, put the corned beef together with whatever spices it came along within the packaging.
- Pour water in the pot until the water is at the same level as the top of the corned beef.
- Cover the Instant Pot and lock the lid. Using MANUAL mode, cook the beef in HIGH PRESSURE with the timer set at 90 minutes. When done, use the quick-release feature of the pot to release the steam.
- Do a doneness test by piercing the beef's thickest area with a fork. If the beef's not easy to pierce with the fork, it means it's undercooked. If so, cook for another 10 minutes.
- Next, place the cabbage wedges and carrots inside the pot. Cover and lock the lid again and using the manual setting, cook for 5 minutes more under high pressure.

– Use the quick release handle to release pressure.
Transfer the corned beef together with the vegetables to
a serving plate. Slice thick pieces of the beef against the
grain and enjoy with cabbage wedges or carrots before
enjoying.

INSTANT POT BUTTER-SAUCED LOBSTER TAILS

This recipe is good for 8 servings with less than 1 gram of carbs per serving.

Ingredients:
- 8 frozen lobster tails;
- 2 teaspoons of lemon juice;
- ½ teaspoon of salt;
- ½ teaspoon of pepper;
- 1 teaspoon of garlic, minced;
- 1 teaspoon of cilantro;
- 1 tablespoon of Old Bay Seasoning (your favorite one);
- 1 cup of water; and
- 1 cup of butter.

Directions:
- Cut a line down the inside of each lobster tail using kitchen shears so you can easily cut even when they're hot.
- Put a cup of water in your 6-quart Instant Pot followed by 1 tablespoon of your favorite Old Bay seasoning.
- Put the trivet at the bottom of your Instant Pot, resting above the water-Old Bay mixture.
- On the trivet, put 4 lobster tails with the side of the shell facing down.
- Put the steamer basket above the first 4 lobster tails on the trivet and on it, place the 4 remaining lobster tails.

- Cover the pot and make sure the vent's setting is on SEALING.
- Press the MANUAL option and set the timer to 4 minutes. Keep in mind that cooking frozen ingredients will extend the pot's heating process, only after which will the pot's timer start counting down from your set steaming time.
- While your lobsters are steaming, you can start making the butter sauce. Cook a tablespoon of butter on a frying pan for 3 minutes or just until it turns brownish. Put the remaining butter in together with 1 teaspoon of freshly minced garlic.
- When the butter has completely melted, throw in the cilantro, pepper, and lemon juice to the mixture. After thoroughly mixing, set the mixture aside.
- When the Instant Pot's timer sounds off, turn the pot off and quickly release the steam, keeping your hands away from the vent out of which steam is released.
- After the pot has completely released all the steam, unlock and open the pot. Use kitchen tongs to remove the lobster tails from the pot to serve with warm with the butter sauce.

If you are enjoying this book, would you be kind enough to leave a review on Amazon because I would like to hear how the book has improved your life. If you make it to the last page of this book and did not enjoy its value, publisher details will be given to inform what could have been done to better serve your expectations.

MEAT POT BALLS

This recipe is good for 5 servings (3 meatballs each) with only 5 grams of carbs per serving.

<u>Ingredients:</u>

For the meatballs:
- 3/4 cup of parmesan cheese, grated;
- 2 tablespoons of chopped parsley;
- 2 eggs;
- 1/4 teaspoons of ground black pepper;
- 1/4 teaspoons of dried oregano;
- 1/4 teaspoon of garlic powder;
- 1/3 cup of warm water;
- 1/2 cup of almond flour;
- 1 teaspoons of kosher salt;
- 1 teaspoons of dried onion flakes; and
- 1 1/2 pounds of ground beef, leaner than 15%.

For Cooking The Meatballs:
- 3 cup of sugar free marinara sauce; and
- 1 teaspoons of olive oil.

<u>Directions:</u>
- Inside a medium-sized bowl, combine all the meatball's ingredients thoroughly with your hands. Create 15 meatballs that are about 2-inches wide each.
- Coat the bottom of your Instant Pot with olive oil. Set to SAUTÉ mode and in it, brown the meatballs. When done, arrange the meatballs in the pot such that in

between meatballs are ½ inch spaces. Don't press the
meatballs down.
- Pour the marinara sauce evenly over the meatballs,
  close and seal the Instant Pot, put it on MANUAL
  mode, choose LOW PRESSURE, and set the timer to 10
  minutes.
- Manually release the steam when the timer sounds off
  by turning the valve. Once the pot's steam has been
  completely released, open the lid and serve the
  meatballs.

POT BEEF STROGANOFF

This recipe is good for 4 servings with 9 grams of carbs per serving.

<u>Ingredients:</u>
- ¾ cup of water;
- ½ to 1 teaspoon of pepper;
- ½ cup of onion, diced;
- 1 teaspoon of salt;
- 1 tablespoon of Worcestershire sauce;
- 1 tablespoon of oil;
- 1 tablespoon of garlic;
- 1 pound of beef stew meat; and
- 1 ½ cups of mushrooms, chopped.

For the finishing:
- ¼ teaspoon of cornstarch to thicken; and
- 1/3 cup of sour cream.

<u>Directions:</u>
- Set the Instant Pot on HIGH pressure and when it's already hot, pour in the oil to heat it. When the oil's already hot, stir-fry the garlic and onions in it for a minute or two.
- Throw everything in save for the sour cream and the cornstarch, close and seal the pot, and continue cooking for 20 minutes on HIGH PRESSURE setting. When done, let the pot naturally release the pressure.

- Open your Instant Pot then switch on the SAUTÉ mode. Throw in the sour cream and mix.
- Mix a slurry of cornstarch with some water then gradually pour it in while continuously stirring the mixture until it becomes thick.
- Remove from the pot and enjoy!

OLIVE LEMON POT CHICKEN

This recipe is good for 8 servings with only 3.1 grams of carbs per serving.

<u>Ingredients:</u>

For The Marinade:
- Juice of 3 lemons;
- 4 tablespoons of extra virgin olive oil;
- 2 sprigs of fresh sage;
- 2 sprigs of fresh rosemary, chopped;
- 2 garlic cloves, chopped;
- 1½ cup of water;
- ¼ teaspoon of pepper;
- ½ bunch of parsley leaves, stems included;
- 1 teaspoon of sea salt; and
- 1 sprig of fresh rosemary, for garnish.

Remaining Ingredients:
- 3 1/2 ounces of Salt-Cured Olives;
- 1/2 cup of dry white wine;
- 1 whole chicken, cut into parts; and
- 1 fresh lemon for optional garnishing.

<u>Directions:</u>
- Make a marinade by finely cutting the garlic, sage, parsley, and rosemary. Mix them together before adding the salt, pepper, lemon juice, and olive oil.

Continue mixing well and when done, set the mixture aside.

- Remove the chicken pieces' skin and set them aside for preparing chicken stock in the future. Put the chicken pieces in a deep dish. Marinate the chicken pieces by pouring the earlier mixture on them until completely covered. Leave them to marinate in the fridge for 4 hours.
- With the cover off, heat up your Instant Pot. When hot, put olive oil (a swirl's worth) in the pot to cook the marinated chicken in until all sides are browned. This may take up to 5 minutes. If you can't cook all the chicken pieces simultaneously due to space constraints in your Instant Pot, do it in batches instead. Put the chicken pieces on a plate and set aside when done.
- De-glaze your cooker by pouring some white wine in it. Let the wine completely evaporate before proceeding further.
- Return the chicken pieces back into the Instant Pot, prioritizing the darker meats (e.g., legs, thighs, and wings) over the lighter-colored meats (e.g., breasts). It's important that the lighter-colored chicken pieces don't touch your Instant Pot's bottom part.
- Pour enough of the marinade on top of the chicken pieces until the marinade level reaches your Instant Pot's minimum liquid level requirement. On average, it should be 1 ½ cups' worth of marinade for most Instant Pot cookers. Add water in case your remaining marinade isn't enough to reach the minimum liquid level of your pot.
- After closing and locking your Instant Pot, cook the chicken at high pressure for 10 minutes. When the timer sounds off, manually release the pressure via the steam release valve and open the pot while keeping the

heat on. Take out the chicken pieces and transfer them to a serving plate that's covered with foil.

- With your pot on medium-high heat with the cover open, let the liquid inside naturally evaporate to only ¼ of its original volume or until it turns thick and syrup-like.
- Reduce the heat to medium-low before returning the chicken pieces back in the Instant Pot to warm them up. Mix and spoon the glaze together with the chicken pieces and allow the pieces to simmer for a few minutes in the glaze before serving. Garnish with rosemary if desired. Just keep in mind that the olives aren't pitted yet!

INSTANT POT CHEESY-TATAS

This recipe is good for 4 servings with only 6 grams of carbs per serving.

<u>Ingredients:</u>
- Up to 1 teaspoon of salt;
- 4 eggs;
- 10 ounces of canned green chilies, diced;
- 1/4 cup of chopped cilantro;
- 1/2 teaspoon of ground cumin;
- 1 cup of shredded cheese, divided; and
- 1 cup of half-and-half.

<u>Directions:</u>
- Beat the eggs, mix the half-and-half in, and combine the diced green chilies, salt, and ½ cup of cheese.
- In a 6-inch pan greased with oil, pour the mixture and cover the pan with an aluminum foil.
- In the Instant Pot, pour 2 cups of water. Then, put a trivet inside.
- Place the pan that's covered with foil on the trivet inside the pot, cover, and seal. Set the Instant Pot to HIGH PRESSURE and set the timer for 20 minutes to cook. After the pot automatically turns off after the set time, allow the pressure to naturally dissipate for 10 minutes, after which release the remaining steam and pressure naturally.
- After removing the foil covering, sprinkle the remaining shredded cheese on top of the cheesy-tata, i.e., the cooked egg mixture. Then, place the pan under a hot

broiler just until the cheese melts, bubbles and turns brown before enjoying.

CHIC-KETO FAUX NOODLE SOUP

This recipe is good for 4 servings with 9 grams of carbs per serving.

<u>Ingredients:</u>
- 6 cups of chicken stock;
- 3/4 cup of chopped green onions;
- 2 tablespoons of virgin coconut oil;
- 2 cups of spiralized daikon noodles;
- 1/8 teaspoon of freshly ground pepper;
- 1/2 teaspoon of dried oregano;
- 1/2 teaspoon of dried basil;
- 1 teaspoon of sea salt;
- 1 pound of chicken thighs, bones and skins removed;
- 1 cup of diced celery; and
- 1 cup of diced carrots.

<u>Directions:</u>
- Sauté the chicken thighs in virgin coconut oil in the inner bowl of your Instant Pot for up to 10 minutes or until they turn nearly cooked through. Afterward, use 2 forks to shred the thighs inside the pot.
- Throw the celery, onions, and carrots in and continue sautéing for 2 more minutes.
- Mix all the remaining ingredients in save for the daikon noodles, cover the pot and seal the lid. Set it on SOUP mode and cook for 15 minutes more.
- When done, throw the daikon noodles in before enjoying.

Conclusion

I hope this book was able to help you to not just learn delicious and easy-to-prepare recipes that are keto-friendly but that it was also able to excite you enough to actually start preparing the recipes and start losing weight on the ketogenic diet. You see, merely "knowing" is just half the battle for losing weight. The other half is "acting" on what you know. As I end this book, I strongly encourage you to start with at least 1 recipe by tomorrow at the latest. After you've tasted how delicious one recipe is, I'm confident that you'll be excited to try out all the recipes in this book – and start losing weight on the ketogenic diet.

Please remember to leave your review on Amazon if you enjoyed this book!

Thank you and always strive to continue growing!

References:

1. https://www.savorytooth.com/instant-pot-chili-verde/
2. https://mariamindbodyhealth.com/instant-pot-reuben-soup/
3. https://www.wholesomeyum.com/recipes/low-carb-buffalo-chicken-soup-recipe/
4. https://whatgreatgrandmaate.com/instant-pot-buffalo-chicken-meatballs/
5. https://www.thenaturalnurturer.com/blog/instant-pot-lemon-garlic-salmon-from-frozen
6. https://www.skinnytaste.com/instant-pot-chicken-cacciatore/
7. https://www.isavea2z.com/pressure-cooker-lobster-tails-butter-sauce/
8. https://twosleevers.com/instant-pot-keto-pork-beef-tips-stroganoff-low-carb/
9. https://www.savorytooth.com/instant-pot-salmon/
10. https://www.ibreatheimhungry.com/instant-pot-meatballs-keto-low-carb/
11. https://twosleevers.com/pressure-cooker-keto-poblano-cheese-quiche/
12. https://www.savorytooth.com/instant-pot-corned-beef-cabbage/
13. https://ketodietapp.com/Blog/post/2016/02/24/keto-oxtail-soup
14. https://www.wholesomeyum.com/recipes/pressure-cooker-chicken-breast-recipe-shredded-chicken/
15. https://alldayidreamaboutfood.com/slow-cooker-low-carb-hungarian-goulash/
16. https://www.skinnytaste.com/honey-teriyaki-drumsticks-skillet-or-instant-pot/

17. https://paleoflourish.com/pressure-cooker-beef-curry-stew-recipe-paleo-keto-lowcarb

18. https://www.healthfulpursuit.com/recipe/low-carb-chicken-noodle-soup/

19. https://inspiralized.com/slow-cooker-boeuf-bourguignon-with-spiralized-vegetables/